The Green Athlete

Eco-Friendly Gear and Training for Sports Enthusiasts

Table of Contents

Chapter 1. Introduction

Dive into our Special Report: The Green Athlete: Eco-Friendly Gear and Training for Sports Enthusiasts, where eco-consciousness combines with the adrenaline of sports. Morning joggers and Olympic athletes alike, let's equip ourselves with sustainable gear and environmentally friendly training habits, to do our part in preserving the beauty of the natural world – our ultimate sports arena. Reading this report will not only reinvent your fitness journey, but also give you the power to make choices that contribute to planet preservation. This isn't just about loving the game, it's about playing it right. Let's revolutionize your sports routine together because going green has never been this thrilling and fulfilling. Are you ready to be the change and embody the spirit of the Green Athlete? Invest in this report and propel yourself into a future of sport where performance meets sustainability!

Chapter 2. The Emergence of the Green Athlete

The environment's health has turned into one of the most pressing issues. From intensive deforestation to escalating pollution, the actions of humanity have significantly harmed the natural world. However, change is well under way, with various sectors incorporating green practices. One area under transformation is the world of sports. Athletes are stepping up, not only on the playing field but also for the environment, thus embodying the concept of the 'Green Athlete.'

2.1. The Transition to Sustainability

The transformation towards being a Green Athlete has been gradual, yet consistent. First largely initiated by environmental enthusiasts who happened to be athletes, they used their platform, reputation, and influence to promote eco-friendly practices. This transition gained momentum, engaging more individuals, organizations, and even the audiences, turning the sports world into a significant player in the fight against climate change. This shift involves adopting sustainable gear and equipment, applying eco-conscious training and fitness habits, and projecting a lifestyle that balances performance with planet preservation.

2.2. Sports Industry: The Carbon Footprint

Sports, in their many manifestations, consume resources and produce waste, contributing to the overall global carbon footprint. From the construction of massive stadiums to the manufacturing of sporting goods, and the energy used to power high-profile events, the sports industry's impact on the environment is significant.

To better understand the scale, consider a single football match. It demands ample energy for stadium lighting, broadcasting equipment, and thousands of spectators' transportation. The food and drink consumed during the game generate substantial waste. However, our Green Athletes are leading the sports industry's transition towards lower carbon emissions by their committed motion towards sustainability.

2.3. Green Athletes: The Vanguard

'Green Athletes' are emerging as environmental stewards within sports. They embody the principle that enhancing performance and endorsing sustainability are not mutually exclusive. Their objective extends beyond winning medals; it also encompasses preserving the environment, leveraging their influence to induce change within the industry and inspire fans.

Athletes such as Lewis Pugh, an endurance swimmer and UN Patron of the Oceans, utilize their platforms to highlight the impacts of climate change. Meanwhile, figures like Olympic ski racer Lindsey Vonn advocate for renewable energy, and NBA star LeBron James is known for his significant investments in sustainable brands. They demonstrate how athletes can be agents of change, prompting significant shifts toward sustainability in sports.

2.4. Green Gear: The Sustainable Transformation

One of the critical aspects of becoming a Green Athlete is the adoption of green gear. Many sports brands are now producing eco-friendly equipment, made from sustainable or recycled materials, thus reducing their carbon footprint. For example, Adidas launched a range of sneakers made from ocean plastic, while Patagonia advocates responsible production through its use of organic cotton and recycled polyester.

Green gear is not only beneficial to the environment but also performs at a high standard, proving that athletes do not have to compromise performance for sustainability. Moreover, through using sustainable sports equipment, athletes actively contribute to a shared vision of a greener future.

2.5. Green Training: Working with Nature

Training is fundamental for any athlete. Traditional methods, though, involve significant energy consumption and waste production, something Green Athletes aspire to change. They embrace routines that balance physical fitness with eco-friendliness, incorporating renewable energy and reducing waste where possible.

Take the instance of solar-powered gyms, where workout practices generate power, an approach also seen in the increasing popularity of outdoor workouts that capitalize on natural environments. Moreover, Green Athletes prefer sustainable hydration and nutrition choices, opting for natural, organic, and local options over excessively packaged or shipped ones.

2.6. The Impact and Implications

The emergence of the Green Athlete signals a progressive shift towards sustainability in the world of sports. These eco-conscious sports individuals are role models and catalysts, inspiring a wide range of audiences, from fans and athletes to organizations and governmental bodies.

Their actions reverberate outwards, influencing not only the games they play, but also the world beyond. Their choices on and off the field transmit a powerful message about the importance of sustainability and the role each person plays in preserving our planet.

Not only this, they are also helping to shape the future of sports – a future where athletes continue to strive for peak performance while ensuring that the planet is not compromised.

The journey of the Green Athlete symbolizes a revolution that celebrates human potential and resilience, married with a deep sense of responsibility towards our planet. It heralds a sports culture that thrives on the adrenaline of sports and the compassion for the natural world. Becoming a Green Athlete is not just about sporting achievement; it's about lending weight to the movement that promises to make the earth a cleaner, greener place – as it rightfully should be.

Chapter 3. Evaluating the Environmental Impact of Conventional Sports Equipment

Sports equipment, a key component in the pursuit of physical fitness, often comes with a hidden environmental cost. Both in production and disposal, many conventional sporting goods leave a striking carbon footprint that profoundly impacts our planet.

3.1. Evaluating the Production Phase

In examining the production phase of traditional sports equipment, we must consider both the raw materials used and the manufacturing processes involved. Many sports require specialized gear, often made from synthetic materials like neoprene, nylon, and polyurethanes, or natural resources like wood and rubber. These materials, while durable and functional, are frequently non-renewable and environmentally demanding to produce.

Neoprene, for instance, is a synthetic rubber primarily used in wetsuits and protective gear, but its production involves the emission of potent greenhouse gases like chloroprene. Similarly, the nylon used in many sportswear items comes from refining crude oil, a fossil fuel with a significant carbon dioxide (CO_2) cost. Polyurethanes, used in various equipment and padding, are derived from oil and gas, two other non-renewable resources.

Likewise, extracting and processing the natural resources used in sports equipment disrupt ecosystems and deplete limited resources.

For instance, using wood for baseball bats, hockey sticks, and other equipment may contribute to deforestation, while the latex extraction for sports balls often involves intensive farming practices that deplete soil nutrients and increase vulnerability to pests and diseases.

The production process itself consumes large amounts of energy. Factories consume power for machining, assembling, and packaging products. Furthermore, the shipment of raw materials and final products involves burning fossil fuels, contributing to CO2 emissions.

3.2. Assessing the Usage Phase

Although the environmental impact during the usage phase of sports equipment is much smaller than the production or disposal phases, it still warrants consideration. The durability of the equipment determines how long it will be in use before needing replacement. High-quality, durable equipment can considerably reduce environmental impact by minimizing the frequency of replacement.

However, conventional sports equipment isn't always designed with longevity in mind. The commercial drive for the latest designs, materials, or technologies can promote a culture of disposability, where equipment is replaced long before it's worn out. This churn of 'in with the new and out with the old' only compounds the environmental issues already associated with the production phase.

Additionally, the care and maintenance required by the equipment during its usage phase can also contribute to environmental costs. For instance, the water and energy used in washing sportswear, the use of cleaning solvents for equipment, or even the electricity required to charge electric sports equipment like treadmills all add up over the lifespan of these products.

3.3. The Disposal Phase and Its Impacts

Disposal is the final stage in the life of sports equipment - but it's far from the least impactful. Both landfilling and incinerating used equipment contribute to pollution.

Most sports equipment is made from mixed materials, making them hard to recycle. For example, tennis balls comprise wool, felt, rubber, and glue, while running shoes often feature a blend of rubber, synthetic fabric, foam, and plastic. Separating and processing these materials for recycling is challenging and energy-intensive. Consequently, many end up in landfills, where they can take hundreds of years to decompose, thereby releasing harmful greenhouse gases such as methane.

Incineration is another common form of disposal for mixed-material equipment. While this process does generate energy, it also produces sizable carbon emissions and can release toxins if not done under precisely controlled conditions.

3.4. The Importance of Life-Cycle Assessments

Given the array of environmental impacts associated with different stages of a sporting item's life, measuring these impacts is crucial. Life-Cycle Assessment (LCA) is a technique that assesses the environmental aspects and potential impacts from cradle (material extraction) to grave (disposal). An LCA considers all stages of a product's life, providing a comprehensive view of the environmental impacts associated with all the life stages of a product.

However, conducting an LCA can be rather complex, given the breadth of the assessment and the need for detailed data.

Nonetheless, with the necessary investment of time and resources, conducting an LCA for sports equipment can yield invaluable insights. These insights can then drive the creation of more sustainable products by identifying phases and aspects with the highest environmental impact and thus, presenting the best opportunities for improvement.

3.5. Towards Sustainable Sports Equipment

Shifting to environmentally friendly practices is the next logical step after quantifying the eco-impact of traditional sports gear. Instead of using non-renewable materials, manufacturers can choose to use alternatives like organic cotton, recycled polyester, or even innovative materials like bioplastics. Additionally, employing renewable energy sources in production processes and utilizing carbon offset programs can significantly lower carbon footprints.

Likewise, consumers can commit to buying second-hand equipment, prioritizing quality over novelty, and properly recycling old gear. Educating themselves about the environmental impact of their purchases is also key.

In summary, evaluating the environmental impact of conventional sports equipment is an important first step in the transition towards a more sustainable sporting world. Green sports is not just a desirable future; it's a necessary one. To ensure the preservation of our natural world - the ultimate playground - we must all become Green Athletes.

Chapter 4. Greenwear: The Revolution of Eco-Friendly Athletic Gear

As the clock strikes dawn, many athletes awaken to a new day of training, grabbing their gear before heading towards their chosen training grounds. Little do they think about the environmental cost their equipment may carry. Yet, recent times have seen a surge in public consciousness towards sustainable living, and this wave has begun to touch athletic gear, coined elegantly as 'Greenwear'.

4.1. The Need for Sustainable Athletic Gear

Sports and athletics have always been about pushing the boundaries, setting new records, and triumphing over trials. However, these endeavours often demand a litany of gear—shoes, clothes, protective padding, and so much more. Traditionally, this equipment has come from harmful, non-renewable, non-biodegradable sources, which, once discarded, linger in landfills, wreaking havoc on the environment. As our understanding of human impact on the environment deepens, the need for sustainability in all aspects of life, including our athletic gear, becomes more apparent.

4.2. The Evolution of Greenwear: From Concept to Reality

The transition from traditional gear to Greenwear represents more than a shift in materials. It is a complete transformation in approach, challenging long-held beliefs about form, function, and performance. But what exactly is Greenwear? At its core, it is about using eco-friendly materials and processes to manufacture sporting goods that meet or exceed their unsustainable counterparts in both performance and durability.

The inception of Greenwear was humble, born out of a need for a planet-friendly lifestyle. Early adopters faced numerous challenges, mostly in terms of performance and strength. However, relentless R&D efforts by eco-conscious athletes, material scientists, and sports goods manufacturers began to change the tide. Today, we have Greenwear that not only rivals traditional gear but often surpasses it.

4.3. Advances in Materials and Fabrication

Greenwear owes its existence to a myriad of revolutionary materials and fabrication methods that minimize environmental impact without compromising athletic performance.

In the realm of clothing, organic cotton, bamboo, and recycled PET (polyethylene terephthalate) stand out. Organic cotton, devoid of toxic pesticides and GMOs used in regular cotton farming, reduces pollution and water wastage, offering a high-performance and breathable alternative for sportswear. Bamboo fabric, besides being sustainable, is antibacterial, making it a perfect choice for sports gear. As for recycled PET, the fabric is strong, water-resistant, and has a significantly lower carbon footprint than virgin synthetic materials.

In the shoes department, we see the use of unique materials. Algae-based foam for instance, brings a biodegradable, equally cushiony alternative to traditional petroleum-based foams. Natural rubber and cork have found their way into inner soles and other parts of athletic shoes.

It's not just the raw materials; progress in fabrication technique has given a push to Greenwear too. Processes like 3D knitting, which reduces waste by creating products that require less cutting and sewing, and waterless dyeing techniques, have contributed significantly to the production of sustainable sports gear.

4.4. Market Success of Greenwear

Choosing Greenwear is no longer a compromise on quality or style, and this is reflected in its market success. Some major sportswear brands have committed to integrating sustainability into their product lines. Though initially met with skepticism, these eco-friendly products have proven highly successful, riding on the back of their performance and a growing global consciousness towards environmental preservation.

Despite being relatively new and ambitious, Greenwear doesn't lag behind when it comes to catering to different sports. You can find eco-friendly alternatives for running gear, yoga wear, swimming suits, cycling shorts, and much more. There's nothing that this bold new world of sustainable sporting gear cannot cater to.

4.5. Embracing Greenwear: A Call to Action

As athletes and sports enthusiasts, it's our responsibility to lead the charge on this front, to make Greenwear the new normal. It's an open field with countless opportunities for improvement and innovation. Adopting Greenwear doesn't just make us better athletes—it makes us better stewards of the planet. Let's seize this opportunity to make an ecological difference, one that will resonate far beyond the boundaries of sports fields and into every aspect of our earth's future.

In conclusion, the transformation towards eco-friendly athletic gear is already underway, driven by innovative new materials, a shift in consumer attitudes, and leading manufacturers' embrace of sustainable practices. The world of athletic gear, traditionally a significant contributor to environmental pollution, is slowly shifting: Going green isn't just possible—it's the future. So gear up with Greenwear, and let's run towards a greener future hand in hand.

Chapter 5. The Rise of Sustainable Sports Brands: Case Studies

In recent years, there has been a growing trend for sustainability in sports brands, with companies increasingly focusing on creating products that are both high-performing and environmentally friendly. Let's dive into the journey of a few pioneers in this sector, their ethos, and their strategies for developing sustainability.

5.1. Sustainable Sports Brands' Ethos

The philosophy behind sustainable sports brands generally aligns with creating high-quality sporting goods without wreaking havoc on the environment during the manufacturing process. Basic principles such as reduction in the use of virgin materials, minimal manufacturing waste, conservation of water and energy, a fair labour-practice environment, and the capacity for reclamation and recycling of used gear are some of the cornerstones of this emerging class of sports brands. Leading companies are determined to push the boundaries, seeking innovative ways to marry high-performance products with underlying environmental responsibility.

5.2. Adidas: Embracing Innovation for Sustainability

Adidas has embraced sustainability as an integral part of its business model. Through a collaborative project with Parley for the Oceans, since 2015, they brought to the market a range of footwear and apparel made partially from recycled ocean plastic.

They famously developed and produced the first performance shoe, assembled with an upper part made entirely from yarn fibers, retrieved from plastic waste, and gill nets recovered from coastal regions. Adidas has set a corporate goal to produce 11 million pairs of shoes containing recycled ocean plastic in 2019.

The company continues to minimize its environmental footprint by expanding its product line, leveraging more renewable energy in manufacturing, and working towards complete recyclability in its product lifecycle.

5.3. Patagonia: Pioneers of an Eco-friendly Outdoors

For many years, Patagonia has been a leader in environmentally conscious sportswear, being one of the first to use recycled materials and organic cotton in its products. As adventurers at heart, Patagonia recognized early on that the natural world – their playground and source of inspiration – was under threat.

Patagonia's 'Ironclad Guarantee' ensures that its gear can be repaired, reused, and, when necessary, recycled. Its Worn Wear program also sells refurbished Patagonia items at a discount, to keep them out of landfills. This brand's perspective on profitability is unique in that it commits to donating a percentage of its proceeds to grassroots environmental groups.

5.4. Puma: Raising the Bar with Sustainable Practices

Puma has taken a unique approach to sustainability, creating an annual Environmental Profit and Loss Account (EP&L) since 2010. This report helps to monetize and measure the environmental impacts of Puma's operations and supply chain, making it easier for the company to identify where it can make improvements.

Puma focuses largely on reducing its water and energy consumption, as well as lowering greenhouse gas emissions. It has launched a line of biodegradable shoes, shirts, and bags, which decompose over time when buried underground, reducing landfill waste.

5.5. Athleta: Empowering Women in Sustainable Fashion

Athleta gives special attention to the issue of sustainability in women's sportswear. The brand aims at bringing the largest possible percentage of sustainable fibers to its entire line, aiming at 80% by the end of 2020.

A certified B Corporation, Athleta is committed to empowering women and girls, reducing its environmental impact, and practising fair trade. It also earned recognition for its efforts towards equal pay and representation, thereby creating a positive social impact along with an environmental one.

5.6. Nike's 'Move to Zero'

Nike has ambitious goals for its contributions to planet preservation, with a mission expressed as a 'Move to Zero' — zero carbon and zero waste.

The company's comprehensive strategy ranges from optimizing its designs to integrating operational efficiency in its global supply chain. It is actively increasing the use of recycled materials in its products and aims for 100% renewable energy usage in its facilities.

The Flyknit shoe line is an example of its sustainable design innovation. Flyknit shoes are engineered to produce 60% less waste than traditional footwear, providing exemplary performance while reducing the environmental footprint.

5.7. A More Sustainable Future in Sports

The adoption of sustainable practices is not a mere marketing gimmick; it is now becoming an integral business model for sports companies worldwide. By incorporating such practices, these brands augur hope for a more sustainable future in sports, thereby creating a positive impact on the environment and transformation within the industry.

The challenges are immense, but these trailblazing companies are demonstrating the possibilities. The convergence of sports with sustainability represents an exciting future – not only in how we play the game but also how we equip ourselves to do so, in a responsible manner. Sustainability in sports gear is not just a trend – it is a movement whose time has come. We, as consumers, are the ones who can drive it.

Chapter 6. Training Green: Modifying Habits for Eco-Conscious Exercise

The inception of eco-conscious exercise assimilates a broader perception of fitness that encompasses both personal and environmental well-being. This outlook necessitates a profound understanding of the concept and significance of eco-consciousness in our daily exercise routine, but also demands perceptible changes in our habits and behaviors. So, today, we plunge into the exploration of how we can modify various facets of our training and incorporate eco-friendly habits into our lives.

6.1. Understanding Eco-Conscious Exercise

Eco-conscious exercise melds physical training with an acute awareness and respect for the environment. The idea behind this approach is to diminish our carbon footprint while pursuing our fitness goals. Modifying our exercise habits not just contributes to preserving the environment but also venture profound benefits which include overall health improvement, better mental health, and saving resources.

6.2. How to Commute Green

The journey to your gym, park, or training facility often constitutes a significant portion of your overall ecological impact. To decrease this, consider cycling or walking if the distance is practical. Not only will this serve as part of your warm-up, but it will also curtail the carbon emissions associated with vehicle use.

For longer commutes, opt to carpool with friends or gym mates. If the option exists, favor public transportation or utilize electric vehicles which have lesser carbon emission than traditional ones. Moreover, consider investing in a home gym or support virtual training programs which can save considerable amounts of commuting energy.

6.3. Choosing the Right Eco-Friendly Training Gear

It's important to consider the environmental impact of the training equipment you use. Opt for eco-friendly alternatives, such as yoga mats made from natural rubber or suits fabricated using recycled materials. On a similar lines, water bottles constructed from stainless steel or glass are better alternatives than those made from plastic.

Additionally, for your athletic attire, prefer organic, recycled, or biodegradable materials. Buying pre-loved sports gear can also contribute in reducing waste, as well as patronizing companies committed to eco-friendly production practices.

6.4. Taking Advantage of Natural Environments

The call of nature provides an array of opportunities for eco-conscious workouts. From a run through the forest to beach volleyball, the natural world unfurls an infinite list of physically and mentally refreshing activities. These cardiovascular workouts not only bring us closer to nature, but they are also energy-efficient—requiring no artificial light or air conditioning.

6.5. Responsible Energy Consumption

Gyms and sports facilities are infamous for high energy consumption due to their significant use of electricity for lighting, heating, and equipment. One way athletes can contribute to reducing this consumption is to train during daylight hours to minimize artificial lighting or choose outdoor workouts.

Selecting gyms equipped with renewable energy solutions, like solar panels, is another excellent way to ensure responsible energy consumption. You can further advocate for energy-efficient appliances and machines in your training facility.

6.6. Water Conservation

Hydration plays an integral role in every fitness routine. However, it's important to ensure this fundamental requirement doesn't contribute to water inefficiency. Rather than using single-use plastic bottles, opt for reusable bottles. If possible, choose showers over baths after your workouts to save water. Advocate for the use of water-saving appliances with your sports facility management.

6.7. Advocacy and Influence

As an athlete, you wield considerable influence, be it among your training peers or on social media. You can use this platform to spread awareness about eco-conscious exercise habits. Encourage your sports facility to undertake environmental initiatives, such as recycling programs or the installation of solar panels.

6.8. Final Thought

The shift to green training is a journey that involves continual learning and adjusting. It entails building awareness, experimentation, and fostering new, sustainable habits – making it not just about the end goals, but the process itself. Indeed, there lies a great deal of empowerment in this knowledge – we hold the power to make a difference, no matter how small or gradual it may seem.

Are you ready to leap into this journey and become a Green Athlete? Remember, every step you take in your training is not only a step towards your individual fitness but also a stride in saving our planet.

The path to eco-conscious exercise, though it requires effort, is both personally and globally rewarding. Start today and experience the fulfillment of uniting personal training with global sustainability. The time has come where performance meets sustainability in the world of sports. It's time for us to step up to the challenge and play our part in this essential change. Because, after all, this isn't just about loving the game, but playing it right!

Remember - there is no Planet B.

Chapter 7. Outdoor Sports: Minimizing Nature Footprint

Outdoor sports can be exhilarating and freeing, inducing a sense of liberation rarely found in mundane, tiled weight rooms. The fresh air rushing past as you run alongside a river, the sun gently gracing your skin as you cycle down a hill, or the serenity of navigating an alpine trail – these experiences are more than just exercises. They're an immersion into stunning panoramas where each breath of crisp, mountain air connects you deeper to the environment.

However, as sports enthusiasts, we have a crucial responsibility to ensure our athletic pursuits don't impair the natural ecosystem. Aiding in the protection of the environment implies integrating sustainable practices into our daily activities. This chapter will serve as your comprehensive guide to minimizing your nature footprint during outdoor sports, focusing on three major sections: sustainable gear, responsible routines, and the promotion of environmentally friendly events.

7.1. Sustainable Gear

From moisture-wicking t-shirts to ultra-light hiking boots, sports gear is essential to any outdoor enthusiast's repertoire. However, the mass production of this equipment often involves non-renewable materials and harmful chemicals, thereby contributing to environmental degradation. Thanks to innovative technology and growing awareness, eco-friendly alternatives are now available that can outright replace, or at least offset, the impact of traditional gear.

When it comes to sustainable clothing, look for garments made from natural or recycled materials. Several brands have been pioneering in this space, using materials like recycled polyester or nylon, organic cotton, and merino wool, all of which possess excellent moisture-management and temperature-regulating properties. Apart from the material, pay attention to the dyeing process. Opt for companies using low-impact, water-conserving methods.

Selection of sustainable footwear includes shoes made out of materials such as natural rubber, cork, and recycled materials. These are breathable, long-lasting, and most importantly, they substantially reduce the carbon footprint compared to conventional counterparts.

For instance, a few brands are producing running shoes with uppers made from recycled ocean plastic or even from coffee grounds. They also focus on using as few materials as possible to make the recycling process easier in the end.

In addition, when choosing equipment like tents, rucksacks, and other essentials, look for those versions made from recycled materials and that don't use harmful chemicals. For example, select tents that are silicone-, PVC-, and fluorocarbon-free to decrease your environmental impact. Choosing gear with long lifespans not only translates to a lower requirement for replacements but also results in less overall waste.

7.2. Responsible Routines

How we conduct ourselves in natural settings is as important as the gear we use. Adopting responsible routines can greatly contribute to minimizing our nature footprint. These routines range from the principles of Leave No Trace to showing respect for local fauna and flora.

Leave No Trace is a set of guidelines developed by the US-based non-profit of the same name. The seven principles are:

1. Plan ahead and prepare

2. Travel and camp on durable surfaces

3. Dispose of waste properly

4. Leave what you find

5. Minimize campfire impact

6. Respect wildlife

7. Be considerate of other visitors

Abiding by these principles involves actions such as sticking to marked trails to prevent erosion and habitat destruction, carrying out all trash, and not removing or disturbing natural features. The sum of our individual actions, no matter how small, greatly influence the conservation of the environments we enjoy.

Moreover, disturbing local fauna and flora could have lasting effects on the balance of the ecosystem. Therefore, observing wildlife from a distance, not feeding animals, and avoiding flora damage are pivotal actions. Awareness and sensitivity towards the environment where we play can go a long way in conserving it for future generations.

7.3. Promoting Environmentally Friendly Events

Transitioning sports events to adopt eco-friendly practices can help to attract new participants who appreciate the efforts being made for environmental protection. Organizers can adopt numerous strategies to make their events more eco-friendly.

In races and tournaments, the move to digital registration and timing systems can save considerable amounts of paper. E-bibs as alternatives to traditional bibs could save tons of non-recyclable material annually.

For refreshment stations, using biodegradable cups and plates, or encouraging athletes to carry their own refillable containers, can curtail plastic waste considerably. Also, collaborating with local food suppliers for catering services can contribute to the local economy and reduce the carbon emissions associated with food transportation.

Promoting carpooling or arranging shared transport for athletes can drastically cut down the carbon emissions produced by these events. In some instances, considering the event location to facilitate public transportation or cycling to the venue can also be a powerful tool in reducing transportation emissions.

Lastly, implementing a proper waste management plan is vital. This could include clearly marked recycling stations for waste segregation, collection of organic waste for composting, and collaborations with specialized companies for the disposal of any residual waste.

Taking action towards minimizing our nature footprint in outdoor sports isn't just about buying green; it's about thinking green and promoting green. This transformation isn't a sprint; it's a marathon, a journey where each decision you make influences the environmental equilibrium. It is on this journey that you'll discover the true essence of being a Green Athlete: understanding the symbiotic relationship between humans and nature, and fully appreciating the playground nature provides.

Chapter 8. Indoor Training and Energy Conservation

In the quest to become a Green Athlete, one can easily overlook the resource consumption that indoor training entails. Yet, the environmental impact of indoor exercise should not be underestimated. Concerns include not only the electricity required to power fitness machines, but also the energy needs of conditioning the indoor environment, and even the manufacture and disposal of equipment. The following guide will delve deeply into these angles, presenting an array of measures for minimizing your carbon footprint within the scope of indoor training, while upholding, and even enhancing, your sporting performance. Moreover, employing the best practices of energy conservation benefits not only the planet, but also your wallet.

8.1. The Energy Footprint of Fitness Equipment

The manufacturing process of sporting goods consumes significant resources, including raw materials and energy. Ideally, a sustainable approach to athleticism dictates the promotion of a "longer life span" philosophy for equipment. Keep your gear well-maintained so they outlast their expected duration, reducing a need for replacement and lessening the impact on our planet's resources. Opting for second-hand equipment is another way to get eco-friendly mileage out of sports gear that would otherwise end up in a landfill.

When buying new equipment, consider the lifespan and energy efficiency of the product. On a treadmill for example, a direct current (DC) motor will generally consume less electricity than the alternative alternating current (AC) motor. Moreover, an efficient design that offers a user-friendly, intuitive interface would likely promote longer treadmill sessions, nourishing both athletic health and equipment longevity.

8.2. Energy-Efficient Conditioning of the Training Environment

Whether it's a home gym, a professional sports complex, or a fitness center, anywhere where physical activity is performed regularly requires specific ambient conditions. Maintaining a certain temperature and air quality involves heating, ventilation, and air conditioning systems (HVAC) which can hog up energy. By employing green HVAC technologies such as geothermal heating or cooling, solar power, and energy recovery ventilators, indoor training areas can significantly lower their contribution to greenhouse gas emissions.

Furthermore, ensure the insulation of your training environment is optimal, to prevent the wastage of energy. Good-quality insulation will hold the required temperature for longer periods, reducing the strain on your HVAC system.

8.3. Implementing Eco-Friendly Lighting

The design and technology of the lighting system have a lasting impact on the energy footprint of a training environment. With indoor training, especially in inclement weather or shorter daylight hours, a well-lit space is indispensable.

Opt for LED lights - they are more energy-efficient and have a longer life-span than traditional incandescent lights. Additionally, consider installing occupancy sensors and timers to ensure lights are used only when necessary.

Natural light and ventilation are another green strategy. Where possible, incorporate windows and skylights into your gym design for a bright, airy space that minimizes electricity consumption.

8.4. Power-Saving Exercise Machines

The bulk of energy consumption in indoor training stems from exercise machines that run on electricity. Treadmills, elliptical trainers, stationary bikes, etc., all require power to function. However, some manufacturers are offering innovative solutions to this problem.

Self-powered machines, like manual treadmills and spin bikes, offer a great way to stay fit while reducing the energy footprint. As the next best alternative, choose equipment adorned with an ENERGY STAR label (or a comparable certificate in your country), which will guarantee significantly lower energy consumption than the average. A unique idea is to invest in equipment that converts physical effort into power - some models of stationary bikes, treadmills, and ellipticals can feed back into the grid or charge a battery.

Remember, every kilowatt saved is a contribution to the environment, making you a true Green Athlete.

8.5. Integrating Power Management Practices

A gym or training facility regularly running dozens of machines often at full power, can amass substantial energy bills. Implementing power management strategies can drastically save energy and cut costs.

One such practice is installing a central power management system. This system ensures all equipment in the facility shuts down or shifts into a power-saving mode during non-operational hours. Encourage individuals to switch off machines and electronic devices when not in use.

Additionally, keep the equipment clean and well maintained. Dust and grime can cause fitness machines to work harder, thus consuming more power.

Finally yet importantly, awareness and education are essential. Encourage and educate all the users of your training facility, be it your family or gym members, about the importance of energy conservation and the role they can play.

Achieving energy efficiency and sustainability in indoor training might seem challenging, but every step you take significantly contributes to protecting the planet. By integrating these practices into your training routines and facilities, you become a torchbearer of the Green Athlete movement, making a difference through sustainable athletic performance.

Chapter 9. Dietary Concerns: Fueling the Green Athlete Sustainably

The age-old adage, "You are what you eat" underscores the correlation between diet and health. For sports enthusiasts striving for peak physical performance while also living an eco-friendly lifestyle, the concept of sustainable eating habits becomes paramount. It encapsulates what, how, and where we eat, all with the aim of reducing our carbon footprints and promoting a healthier planet.

9.1. Understanding Sustainable Eating Habits

Sustainable eating habits revolve around food choices that not only fit your macro and micronutrient needs but also have minimal impact on the environment. They are built on the principle of consuming foods produced, processed, and distributed in ways that are healthier for our planet as well as our bodies.

Here's a starter list of sustainable food choices:

- Choose organic: Organic foods are grown free from synthetic fertilizers and pesticides, and they adhere to standards designed to preserve biodiversity, sustain productivity, and promote ecological balance. Evidence shows that organic farming methods can reduce carbon emissions into our atmosphere.

- Opt for fair-trade: Choosing fair-trade products helps support responsible companies, cultivates environmental stewardship, and bolsters sustainable farming practices globally.

- Eat locally: Locally grown and sourced foods reduce emissions resulting from transporting food over long distances. They also support local economies and farming industries.

- Consider seasonal food: Like locally sourced foods, seasonal foods reduce the need for energy-intensive greenhouses and long-distance transportation.

9.2. Optimizing Your Athlete Plate

Regardless of the source, food fuels our bodies providing the energy and nutrients necessary to perform. The athletes' plate should be a well-balanced mix of macronutrients - carbohydrates, proteins, and fats - and micronutrients - vitamins and minerals.

Carbohydrates, the primary energy source for athletes, should comprise about 45-65% of total calorie intake. Whole-grain products, fruits and vegetables, beans, and legumes provide high-quality, fiber-rich carbohydrates. Proteins, essential for muscle growth and repair, should be approximately 10-35% of total calories. Lean sources of animal protein, such as poultry, fish, and dairy, along with plant-based proteins, can fulfill protein needs. Fats, needed for energy reserves, should make up 20-35% of daily calorie intake. Unsaturated fats from sources like avocados, nuts, seeds, and olive oil are healthful choices.

However, these numbers might fluctuate based on the type of sport, intensity level, training schedule, gender, and individual goals. Food should be consumed in smaller portions several times a day versus a few larger meals to continually replenish nutrients and sustain energy levels.

9.3. Upholding the Principle of Hydration

Staying hydrated is crucial for any physical activity. Dehydration can lead to disturbances in muscular function and strength due to the lack of water needed for energy reactions. Plain water works as the best source of hydration. Always avoid plastic bottled water; instead, opt for reusable bottles. For higher-intensity sports or longer training sessions, sports drinks abundant in electrolytes can be added.

9.4. Supplements: A Sustainable Path?

Nutritional supplements are often seen in the world of sports. While some may be beneficial, an over-reliance on supplements versus whole foods can overlook the importance of diversity in diet. It's best to consider supplements only when a balanced diet does not meet nutritional needs or in certain conditions advised by a dietitian. From a sustainability perspective, choosing brands that invest in recyclable packaging or source nutrients responsibly can contribute to your eco-friendly journey.

9.5. Managing Waste and Recycling

Once we have food sourcing, meal planning, and a balanced diet in check, the next concern is waste management. Lessening food waste involves meal planning, using leftovers creatively, and composting. Meanwhile, recycling should become habitual, including proper sorting of recyclable materials like glass, plastics, and metals.

9.6. Meal Planning for Athletic Performance

A well-planned meal strategy helps align your dietary choices to both sports performance goals and sustainability principles. Start with setting up a weekly meal plan, incorporating a balanced distribution of macronutrients in each meal. Plan your food shopping to reflect your meal plan, focusing on package-free, organic, and locally sourced items when possible.

Ultimately, the green athlete's journey to sustainable fueling might appear challenging initially, but the cumulative effects of these daily choices have considerable potential. Implementing sustainable eating habits will not only aid you in achieving your athletic goals but will also embrace the larger picture of ecological well-being, embodying the ethos of a true Green Athlete. It should not be viewed as a trade-off but rather an integration of performance and planet preservation, making us all winners in the grand arena of life.

Chapter 10. Community and Networking: Green Sports Events and Organizations

The advent of Green Sports Events and Organizations has blurred the boundaries between individualistic pursuits for athletic prowess and collective eco-conscious responsibilities. Emphasizing on the shift towards sustainability in sports, this chapter will unravel the various dimensions of the role communities and networking plays in the sphere of green athletics.

10.1. Eco-Friendly Sports Events: The Green Revolution

One can't talk about sustainability and sports without dwelling into the significant role played by environmentally friendly sports events. These events are often the intersection of environmental philanthropy, conscious consumption, community participation, and athletic commitment. Gone are the days when professional sports events catapulted only the most exceptional athletes into the limelight. Now, these events are platforms for a broader community to rally behind shared beliefs and concerns, particularly about environmental conservation.

Imagine a marathon where all participating athletes wear shirts made from recycled material, where the hydration stations serve refreshments in biodegradable cups, and the energy consumed by the event comes from renewable sources. Suddenly, the marathon manifesto doesn't merely talk about resilience and endurance; it extends to consider the preservation of the planet too. Many sports festivals like the Coachella Valley Music and Arts Festival and the Bonnaroo Music and Arts Festival have already begun making decisive moves towards the green direction.

Such sporting events make a significant impact on their audiences, urging competitors and spectators alike to reflect on their environmental footprints. By exposing attendees to green practices, they are setting the stage for a more eco-conscious society.

10.2. Network of Green Organizations: Guardians of Green Sports

Along with the growing consciousness about our planet's health, we've seen the emergence of green organizations committed to promoting sustainable practices in the sports industry. The Green Sports Alliance and Biodegradable Sports Gear (BSG) are examples of such organizations that are tirelessly working to ensure a smooth transition to green sports.

With a vast community of sports leagues, teams, fans, and environmentally focused partners, the Green Sports Alliance leverages the cultural and market influence of sports to promote healthy, sustainable communities where we live and play. They advise sports organizations on how to adopt green practices, hold sports events with minimal carbon footprint, and encourage the consumption of eco-friendly sports gear.

BSG, on the other hand, offers sustainable alternatives to conventional sports gear. They sell items made from biodegradable materials and other environment-friendly components. BSG partners with local sports teams and organizations, driving the adoption of green sports practices and gear.

10.3. Crowdfunding and Sponsorships

Crowdfunding and sponsorships play a significant role in mitigating the additional costs that come with promoting sustainable sports events and eco-friendly athletic gear. Platforms like Kickstarter and GoFundMe have become popular spaces for green athletes and event organizers to raise funds.

Several sponsors are also keen on supporting environmentally friendly events since showing support for sustainability often augments their brand image. Many businesses understand that aligning with environmental causes can help them reach a broader customer base who appreciates and supports these values, thereby making sponsorships a win-win for both parties.

10.4. Fans: Integral Part of the Green Movement

Fan communities can significantly enhance the impact of green sports initiatives. The more the fans support teams or athletes who strongly advocate for sustainability, the broader the reach of the message. By buying merchandise made from recycled materials, consuming food and drink from sustainable sources at games, or using public transportation to reach the sporting venues, fans become an indispensable part of this green revolution.

10.5. Educating the Masses

Community outreach and education are essential aspects of the green sports movement. It's critical to educate the masses about the importance of sustainable sports practices. Sports organizations and green athletic advocates can conduct workshops, set up green exhibits at events, or use social media platforms to share information and tips.

In conclusion, green sports events and organizations have embraced the power of community and networking to create a broader impact. These collective efforts are not only revolutionizing the future of sports but are also setting the stage for a more sustainable world. As we navigate this journey, every athlete, fan, and sports enthusiast becomes part of the solution, reinventing the world of sports as we know it.

Chapter 11. The Future of Sports: Predictions and Opportunities for Sustainable Innovation

As we look towards the horizon, it's clear that the future of sports is anchored in sustainable innovation. Advancement in both technology and eco-awareness have presented us with ample opportunities to fundamentally transform the sports industry, from manufacturing equipment to athletes' training routines. This transition treads a path that intertwines performance with environmental responsibility, propelling us into a new era—a future of sports where excellence is measured not only by points and seconds, but also by our ability to reduce our ecological footprint.

11.1. Traditional Sports and Environment: A Retrospective

The sports industry has historically had a significant environmental impact. From energy-intensive stadiums, use of synthetic materials in gear, to high fuel consumption for intercontinental tournaments, sports events, big or small, have left conspicuous footprints on the environment. However, reflecting on these practices isn't about condemning them but about understanding the necessity for a greener shift.

11.2. Opportunities for Sustainable Innovations

From energy-efficient infrastructures to eco-friendly sportswear, the sports industry is bestowed with opportunities for sustainable innovations.

11.2.1. Eco-friendly Sporting Goods

The innovation in eco-friendly sports equipment has been remarkable. Many companies are incorporating sustainable materials into their products, such as recycled packaging or ethically sourced raw materials. These sustainable processes not only reduce waste but also set an example for other industries to follow.

Notably, sports apparel has seen a greener transformation. Brands like Adidas have launched product lines made from recycled ocean plastics, while others like Patagonia have committed to ethical and sustainable manufacturing practices. This trend is only the beginning, and the foreseeable future envisages a surge in eco-friendly sports gear availability.

11.2.2. Greener Infrastructure

Sports infrastructure, especially stadiums and athletic training facilities, consumes vast amounts of energy. There's an emerging need for energy-efficient sports infrastructure, ranging from the use of renewable sources like solar panels to LED lights and water recycling systems.

An excellent example of this is the Sacramento Kings' Golden 1 Center, the world's first LEED Platinum indoor sports arena, powered entirely by solar energy. NFL's Atlanta Falcons' Mercedes-Benz Stadium is another precedent of sustainable design that harvests rainwater to prevent flooding. Change has begun, but it needs to become the norm rather than an exception.

11.3. Breakthrough Technology and Innovations

Technological breakthroughs are instigating a transformative wave in sustainable sports practices.

11.3.1. Virtual Reality (VR) Training

Virtual reality is emerging as an eco-friendly training tool. It eliminates the need to travel, reducing greenhouse gas emissions associated with transportation. From running scenic trails from your living room to practicing match situations in soccer or cricket, VR opens up new possibilities for eco-friendly sports training.

11.3.2. Data Analytics and AI

Data analytics and AI are empowering sports industry to become more sustainable by optimizing resource usage and improving waste management. Software solutions can now track the usage patterns of energy, water, and other resources in sports facilities. These insights can be used to adjust systems to run more efficiently, drastically reducing carbon footprints.

11.4. The Post-Pandemic Sports: An Indirect Push Towards Sustainable Practices

The COVID-19 pandemic indirectly catalyzed the urgent need for sustainable practices. With the disturbance in international trade and increased skepticism in international travel, local sourcing has caught momentum, a development that has lower environmental impact.

11.5. The Athlete's Role: Pioneers for a Sustainable Future

Athletes have a unique role as influencers and advocates for sustainable sports. Some athletes are already using their platform to raise awareness, such as the NBA's eco-activist, Malcolm Brogdon, who is advocating for the use of renewable energy. The more athletes engage in the sustainability dialogue, the more momentum the movement gains.

11.6. The Fan's Role: Supportive Sports Consumers

Fans are not bystanders but play an essential role in the transition. Through supportive consumption of sustainably produced sports gear, preferentially attending eco-friendly sports events, and demanding corporations to adopt greener practices, fans can really drive the change.

In conclusion, the future of sports with sustainable innovation appears promising, ripe with numerous opportunities. It is not a question of 'if' but 'when' and 'how' the broad adoption of these practices will occur. An environmentally friendly revolution is on the horizon in the sports world, heralding a future where the ecstasy of victory aligns harmoniously with the preservation of our planet's resources.

www.ingramcontent.com/pod-product-compliance
Lightning Source LLC
Chambersburg PA
CBHW071038260726
48661CB00007B/3046